Keto Friendly Cocktails

Easy Low Carb Recipes from Negroni and Old Fashioned to Skinny Margarita and Long Island

Jenny Kern

Table Of Contents

Introduction

Thank you for purchasing this book.

The most common way to prepare cocktails and most other drinks too is the Building. When using this method, all the ingredients are poured directly and mixed into the glass in which they are to be served. This is the method you will use whenever you see "build in the glass" or something similar in a recipe in the book. In this book you will learn how to make different cocktails with various techniques. I am sure you will create some fabulous drinks.

Enjoy.

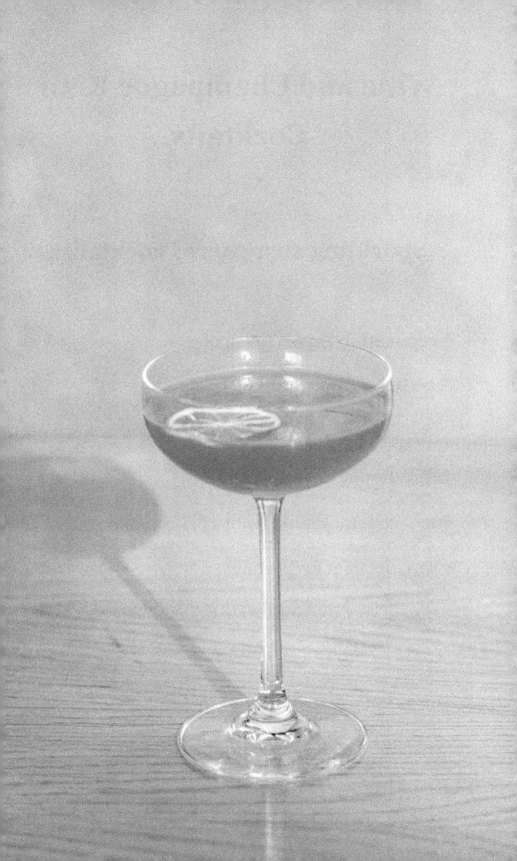

Wine and Champagne Keto Cocktails

Sparkling strawberry cocktail

Preparation time: 10 minutes

Servings: 2

Ingredients:

8 medium strawberries with a perfect shape

2 sprigs of mint to decorate

6.8oz. of very cold Italian sparkling wine

Directions:

Clean, wash and dry the strawberries gently.

Distribute them in the glasses you have chosen.

Pour the wine equally into the two glasses.

Decorate with mint and serve immediately.

Tips:

Avoid strawberries that are not very fragrant.While if you find them, you can use wild strawberries.

Mandarin and pomegranate cocktail

Preparation time: 10 minutes

Servings: 1

Ingredients:

8 mandarins

brut sparkling wine

half of a pomegranate

Directions:

Squeeze the mandarin and filter the juice with a very thick sieve.

Collect the juice in a very large carafe. Take the pomegranate seeds and add them to the jug. Finally, pour the sparkling wine, mix well and serve.

As an alternative to tangerines, you can use both clementines. The sparkling wine can instead be replaced with champagne or Prosecco. But they must be cold.

Then decorate the glass with slices of mandarin or wedges peeled and cut in half.

Cocktail with kiwi and sparkling wine

Preparation time: 15 minutes

Servings: 2

Ingredients:

2 kiwis

2 tablespoons of dry sparkling wine

1 orange

2 tablespoons of gin

Directions:

Put a glass in the freezer so that it is well cooled when needed. Put the sparkling wine in the fridge and, in the meantime, peel the kiwis and cut them into cubes. Wash the orange and remove some zest with the Zester.

Squeeze the orange and collect the juice in a bowl, then filter it and put it in the blender glass with the diced kiwis and the gin, blend 3 minutes at medium speed.

Put the smoothie in the glass and complete by stretching with the cold sparkling wine, decorate with the orange peel strips, and serve immediately.

Strawberry cocktail

Preparation time: 15 minutes

Servings: 4

Ingredients:

1 small basket of strawberries

dry sparkling wine to taste

Directions:

Gently wash and dry the strawberries, and set aside one for each glass for the final decoration, and remove the stalk from the others.

Put the strawberries inside the mixer, blend them, and then pass the smoothie obtained through a colander to eliminate the seeds.

Put it in the fridge for 30 minutes.

Pour the smoothie into the glasses, filling it 1/3, then add the dry sparkling wine, filling it 2/3, and mix.

Put a whole strawberry in each glass, then serve the cocktail.

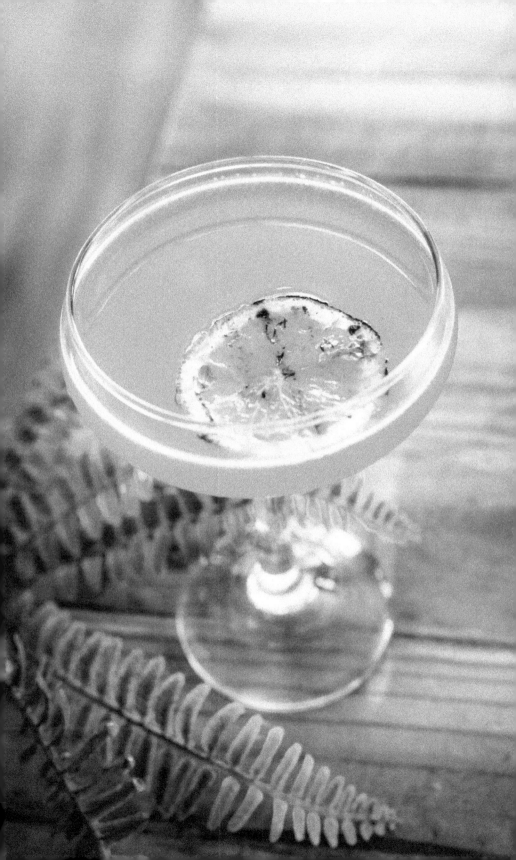

Gin Keto Cocktails

Rhubarb Gin

Preparation time: 10 minutes

Servings: 2

Ingredients:

400 g (14 oz.) caster sugar

1 kg (35 oz.) pink rhubarb stalks

800 ml (27 oz.) gin

Directions:

Wash the rhubarb, trim the stalks and get rid of the base and all leaves.

Cut the rhubarb stalks into pieces and put them in a big jar with the sugar.

Shake everything and leave to rest overnight.

After about 24 hours, you can add the gin and shake the mixture once again.

Leave to rest for at least 4 weeks before serving.

Pink Negroni

Preparation time: 10 minutes

Servings: 2

Ingredients:

35 ml (1.2 oz.) pink gin

15 ml (0.5 oz.) Aperol

25 ml (0.85 oz.) rose vermouth

Ice cubes

Some wedges of pink grapefruit, to garnish

1 basil leaf, to garnish

Directions:

Pour the Aperol, pink gin, and vermouth in a tumbler along with ice. Stir well.

Add some pink grapefruit wedges and a basil leaf to garnish, before serving.

Aviation

Preparation time: 10 minutes

Servings: 2

Ingredients:

1½ oz. gin

¾ oz. Maraschino liqueur

¼ oz. violet liqueur

½ oz. lemon juice

Ice

Lemon zest, for garnish

Directions:

Pour ½ oz. of lemon juice, ¾ oz. of Maraschino liqueur, ¼ oz. of violet liqueur, and 1½ oz. of gin

Fill the glass with ice cubes and stir gently

Garnish with lemon zest after straining in a chilled glass

Clover Club

Preparation time: 5 minutes

Servings: 1

Ingredients:

1½ oz. gin

1 oz. raspberry syrup

½ oz. lime juice

1 egg white

Ice

3 raspberries, for garnish

Directions:

Pour 1 egg white, ½ oz. of lime juice, 1 oz. of raspberry syrup, and 2 oz. of gin into a shaker

Fill the shaker with ice cubes and shake thoroughly

Garnish with three raspberries after straining in a chilled glass

Bramble

Preparation time: 10 minutes

Servings: 2

Ingredients:

1½ oz. gin

½ oz. crème de mûre

½ oz. sugar syrup

¾ oz. lime juice

Raspberry

Crushed ice

1 slice of lemon

Directions:

Place 4 raspberries into rocks glass and muddle

Fill the glass to the top with crushed ice

Pour in ¾ oz. of lemon juice, ½ oz. of sugar syrup, and 1½ oz. of gin and stir gently

Top up with crushed ice

Pour over ½ oz. crème de mûre

Garnish with a raspberry and a slice of lemon

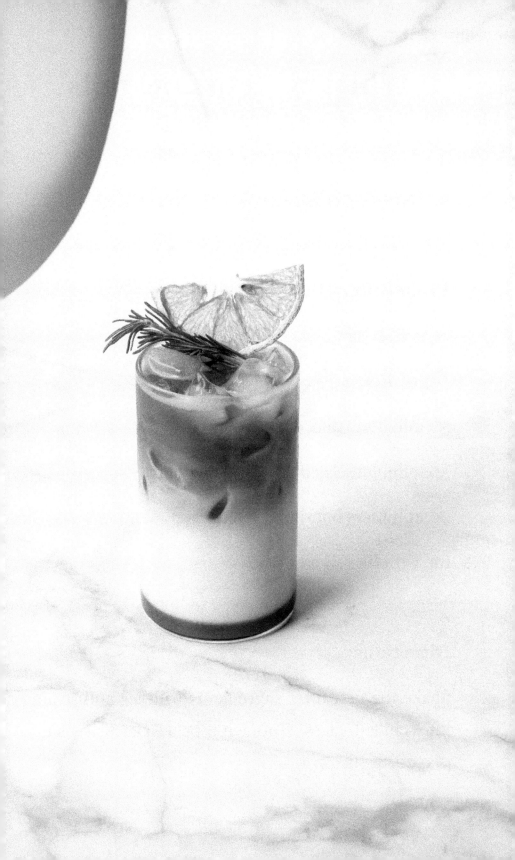

Whiskey Keto Cocktails

Swedish Spear

Preparation time: 10 minutes

Servings: 2

Ingredients:

30 milliliters pink grapefruit juice

30 milliliters Swedish punsch liqueur

60 milliliters bourbon whiskey

top with British bitter ale

Directions:

Shake the first three ingredients with ice and strain into chilled glass. Top with beer. Garnish using grapefruit slices.

Steel Petal

Preparation time: 10 minutes

Servings: 2

Ingredients:

15 milliliters absinthe

1 dash Peychaud's Bitters

30 milliliters Amaro liqueur

30 milliliters Aperol Aperitivo

45 milliliters rye whiskey

Directions:

Rinse mixing glass with absinthe. Stir the rest of the ingredients with ice and strain into chilled glass. Garnish using orange zest twist.

Soul Thrust

Preparation time: 10 minutes

Servings: 2

Ingredients:

4 milliliters Pedro Ximénez sherry

8 milliliters Islay whiskey

8 milliliters walnut liqueur

22 milliliters sweet vermouth

45 milliliters blended scotch whiskey

2 dashes whiskey barrel-aged bitters

Directions:

Stir ingredients with ice and strain into chilled glass.
Garnish using orange zest twist.

Snake Pit

Preparation time: 10 minutes

Servings: 2

Ingredients:

45 milliliters bourbon whiskey

45 milliliters dry vermouth

45 milliliters pink grapefruit juice

Directions:

Shake ingredients with ice and strain into chilled glass. Garnish using lemon zest twist.

Classic Hot Toddy

Preparation time: 5 minutes

Servings: 2

Ingredients:

3 tsp honey, runny honey works best with this cocktail

50ml whiskey

The juice of one lemon

A few lemon slices for decoration

2 cloves

200ml boiling water

1 halved stick of cinnamon

Directions:

Take a small mixing jug and combine the honey and the whiskey

Take two glasses, heatproof, and add a cinnamon stick half to each

Add 100ml of boiling water to each glass

Divide the lemon juice between the glasses

Decorate each glass with lemon slices and one clove in each

Serve whilst still hot

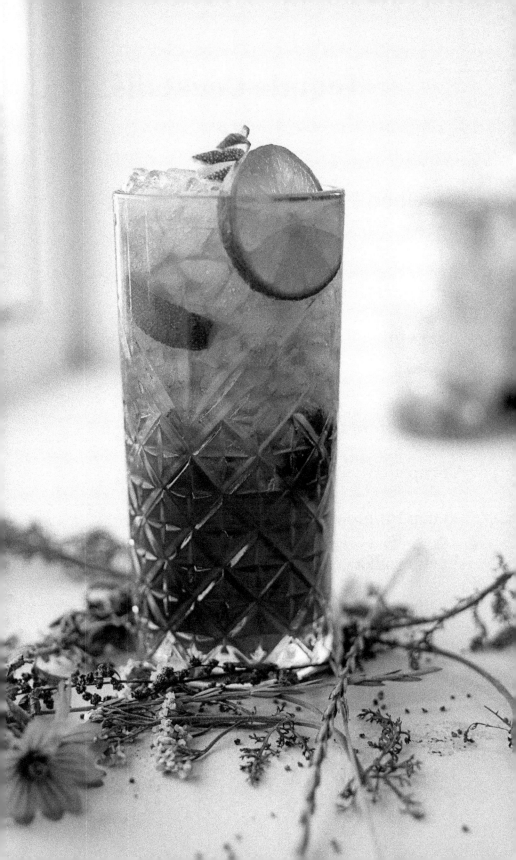

Tequila Cocktails

Coco Lopo

Preparation time: 15 minutes

Servings: 8

Ingredients:

1 cup gin

1 cup 151 proof rum

1 cup vodka

1 cup tequila

1 cup grenadine syrup

1 (8 ounce) can cream of coconut

Directions:

Pour the gin, rum, vodka, tequila, grenadine, and cream of coconut into a blender; fill with ice; blend until smooth.

Coconut Margarita

Preparation time: 10 minutes

Servings: 8

Ingredients:

2 cups sweet and sour mix (such as Bone Daddy®)

1 cup tequila (such as Cuervo Gold®)

1/2 cup triple sec liqueur

1/2 cup coconut milk

2 limes, juiced

Directions:

Mix sweet and sour mix, tequila, triple sec, coconut milk, and lime juice in a pitcher, stirring vigorously. Serve over ice.

Coronarita

Preparation time: 10 minutes

Servings: 2

Ingredients:

2 (12 fluid ounce) cans or bottles lemon-lime soda, or more to taste

1 (12 ounce) bottle of Mexican beer (such as Corona®)

1 (12 fluid ounce) can frozen limeade concentrate

12 fluid ounces tequila

Ice

2 leaves mint, chopped, or more to taste (optional)

Directions:

Pour lemon-lime soda, Mexican beer, and frozen limeade into a large pitcher. Use an empty limeade can to measure out tequila; pour into the pitcher. Mix well to combine. Serve over ice garnished with chopped mint.

Cowboy Margaritas

Preparation time: 10 minutes

Servings: 6

Ingredients:

1 (12 ounce) container frozen limeade concentrate

6 fluid ounces tequila

3 fluid ounces raspberry-flavored liqueur

1 (12 fluid ounce) can or bottle light beer

Directions:

Blend limeade, tequila, and raspberry-flavored liqueur in a blender until well mixed. Slowly stir light beer into limeade mixture.

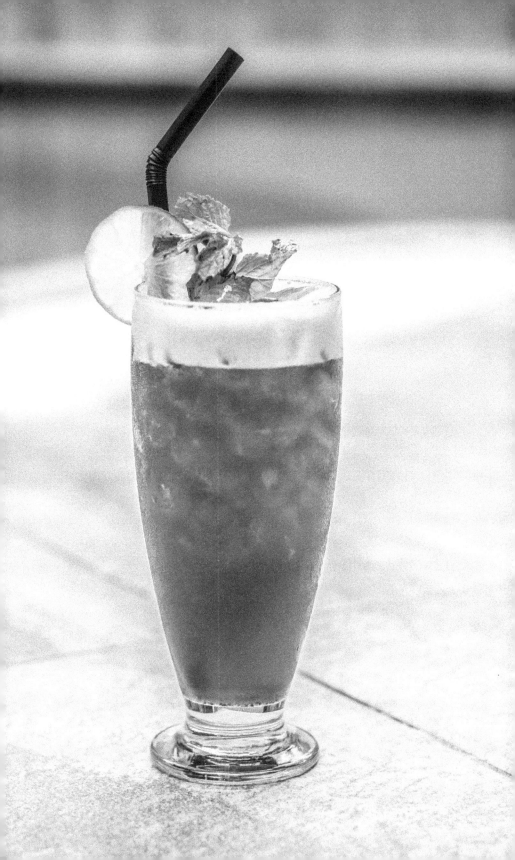

Rum Keto Cocktails

Zesty Berry Punch

Preparation time: 10 minutes

Servings: 6

Ingredients:

350ml rum, dark rum works best with this recipe

1 liter of chilled cranberry juice

1 liter of chilled ginger ale

Ice cubes

Directions:

Take a large punch bowl and pour the cranberry juice and ginger ale inside, stirring until combined

Pour the rum into the bowl and combine once more

Pour into cocktail glasses and top with plenty of ice cubes

Boozy Coconut Punch

Preparation time: 5 minutes

Servings: 2

Ingredients:

250ml rum, Malibu is a good choice for this coconut-based cocktail

500ml fresh pineapple juice

500ml fresh mango juice

250ml tinned coconut milk

A handful of ice cubes

A few slices of pineapple for decoration

Directions:

Take a large mixing jug and add the ingredients together, combine well

Add some ice to each glass

Pour the punch into each glass

Decorate with a slice of pineapple

Spicy Rum 75

Preparation time: 10 minutes

Servings: 6

Ingredients:

200ml rum

600ml champagne, you could use Prosecco if you can't find champagne

60g caster sugar

30ml water

1 tbsp ground allspice

90ml fresh lime juice

A few slices of orange for decoration

Directions:

Take a small saucepan and add the sugar, water, and the allspice

Stir gently over medium heat until the sugar has completely dissolved

Remove the pan from the heat and allow to completely cool

Once cooled, use a fine sieve to remove any grains of allspice from the mixture

Take a cocktail shaker and add the rum, lime juice, and the strained spice mixture

Combine the mixture by shaking vigorously

Take 6 champagne flutes and divide the mixture evenly between, leaving a little space at the top

Top up the glasses with the champagne or Prosecco

Decorate with a slice of orange

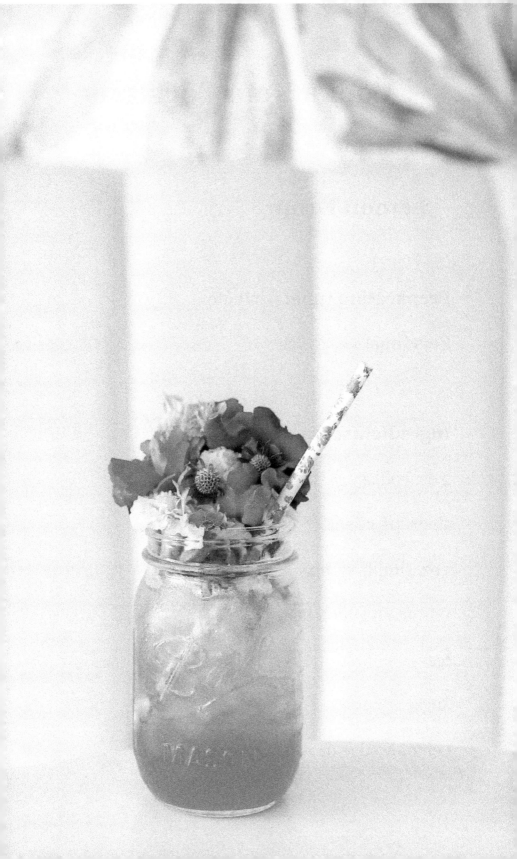

Vodka Keto Cocktails

Lemon Drop

Preparation time: 5 minutes

Servings: 1

Ingredients:

2 oz. vodka

1/2 oz. triple sec

1 oz. simple syrup

1 oz. fresh lemon juice

Ice

Sugar

Lemon wedge or zest, for garnish

Directions:

Add all the ingredients into a shaker with ice and shake.

Coat the rim of a cocktail glass with sugar and set it aside.

Pour into the glass.

Garnish with a lemon wedge or zest.

Rosé All Day

Preparation time: 10 minutes

Servings: 6

Ingredients:

1 bottle of rosé

½ cup vodka

4 ½ cups blackberry sparkling water

1 tablespoon fresh lime juice

2 tablespoons honey

¾ cup blackberries

1 lime, sliced

½ cup raspberries

½ cup strawberries, sliced

Ice

Directions:

Pour ingredients into a pitcher and gently stir until combined.

Pour into your serving glasses and top with fruits.

Vodka Mojito

Preparation time: 10 minutes

Servings: 6

Ingredients:

11/2 mint syrup

1 cup vodka chilled

¼ cup fresh lime juice

1 cup club soda chilled

Ice

Fresh mint sprigs

1 cup water

1 packed cup fresh mint leaves

Directions:

Mix the lime juice, club soda, vodka, and simple syrup. Pour it into a glass filled with ice and garnish it with mint.

Take mint leaves, water and sugar then place the mix over a heated saucepan

Boil the mix while stirring until the sugar dissolves then cool the syrup for ten minutes.

Kamikadze

Preparation time: 10 minutes

Servings: 5

Ingredients:

1½ oz. vodka

1 oz. triple sec liqueur

1 oz. lime juice

Ice

Lime wedge or zest, for garnish

Directions:

Pour 1 oz. of lime juice, 1 oz. of triple sec liqueur, and 1½ oz. of vodka into a shaker

Fill the shaker with ice cubes and shake

Garnish after straining in a chilled glass

Highball glass Martini With a Passion Fruit Twist

Preparation time: 10 minutes

Servings: 3

Ingredients:

60ml vanilla flavored vodka

1 tbsp fresh lime juice

1 tbsp sugar syrup

30ml quality Passoa

2 passion fruits, cut into halves

Prosecco for serving

A handful of ice cubes

Directions:

Prepare the passion fruit by removing the seeds and the skin, keeping the seeds to one side

Take a cocktail shaker and add the seeds

Add the Passoa, vodka, sugar syrup, and the lime juice

Add a few ice cubes

Give the shaker a good shake

Use a strainer to pour the drink into two martini-style glasses

Add a little Prosecco to the top

Add half a passion fruit to each glass

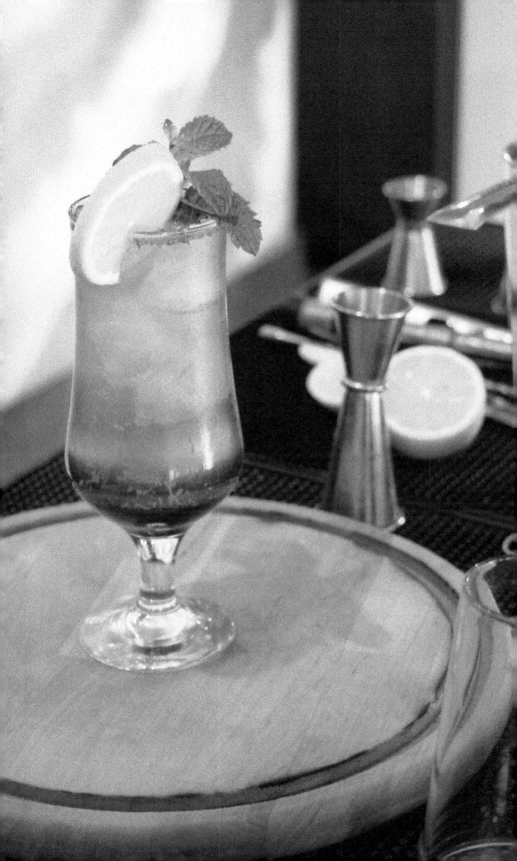

Keto Liqueurs

Bikini Martini

Preparation time: 10 minutes

Servings: 3

Ingredients:

8 milliliters lemon juice

8 milliliters peach schnapps liqueur

15 milliliters cold water

22 milliliters blue curaçao liqueur

60 milliliters London dry gin

Directions:

Shake ingredients with ice and strain into chilled glass. Garnish using orange zest twist.

Biscotti Spritz

Preparation time: 5 mins

Servings: 1

Ingredients:

30 milliliters butterscotch liqueur

30 milliliters hazelnut liqueur

90 milliliters sparkling wine

top with soda

Directions:

Pour sparkling wine and liqueur into the glass. Put in ice. Top with soda. Serve with biscotti.

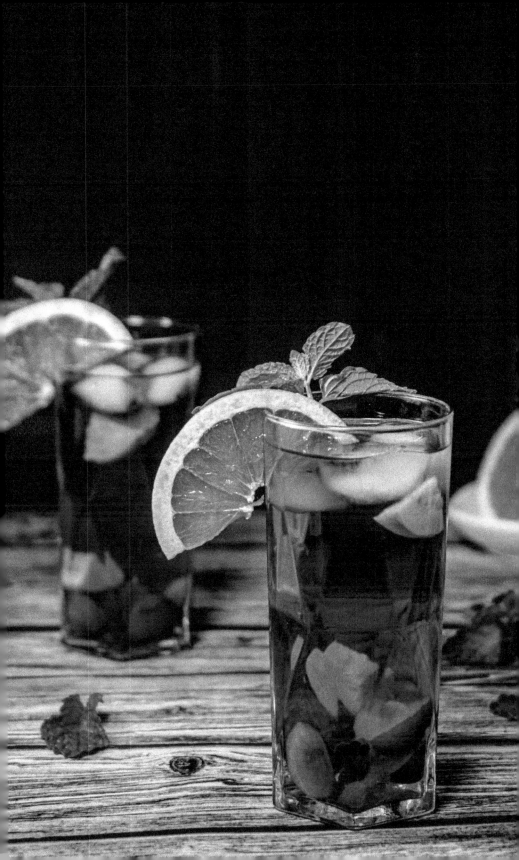

Keto Mocktails

Raspberry Lime Fizz

Preparation time: 10 minutes

Servings: 4

Ingredients:

1 cup raspberries, fresh or frozen, thawed if frozen

Additional 1 cup raspberries, frozen

3/4 cup sugar

5 cups (40 ounces) cold club soda

½ cup fresh lime juice (9 to 10 limes)

Crushed ice

Directions:

Process raspberries in a blender until pureed; strain to remove seeds and pulp.

In a pitcher, combine raspberry juice, sugar, club soda, and lime juice. Stir to combine; taste and add more sugar if desired.

Serve over ice, spooning a few frozen raspberries into each glass.

Watermelon-Lime Slushie

Preparation time: 10 minutes

Servings: 4

Ingredients:

3 cups chopped fresh watermelon

1 tablespoon sugar or natural sugar substitute

1 cup crushed or shaved ice

2 tablespoons fresh lime juice (1 to 2 limes)

½ cup water or lemon-lime soda

Watermelon wedges; garnish; optional

Directions:

Place all ingredients in a blender and process until smooth. Taste, adjust sugar and lime juice if desired, and serve immediately, garnished with watermelon wedges if desired.

Icy Arnold Palmer

Preparation time: 10 minutes

Servings: 4

Ingredients:

4 single-serving size bags of black tea

4 cups boiling water

1 cup water

1 cup sugar

1 cup fresh lemon juice (8 to 10 large lemons)

2 cups crushed ice

Directions:

In a heat-safe pitcher, pour boiling water over tea bags and allow to steep for 5 minutes. Place in the refrigerator.

In a medium saucepan, combine 1 cup water and sugar; cook over medium heat until sugar is dissolved. Cool completely.

Add sugar syrup, lemon juice, and ice to a blender; process until a slushie consistency is reached.

Remove pitcher from refrigerator; add lemonade slush mixture and stir to combine. Taste and add more sugar if desired. Serve immediately.

Note:

To serve a crowd, you can prepare our Southern Iced Tea and Classic Lemonade recipes and combine them in a punch bowl or several large pitchers.

Rosemary Mint Lemonade

Preparation time: 10 minutes

Servings: 4

Ingredients:

½ cup sugar

½ cup water

2 tablespoons fresh rosemary leaves

2 tablespoons fresh mint leaves

1 cup fresh lemon juice (8 to 10 large lemons)

3 cups water

Additional fresh rosemary and mint (for garnish; optional)

Directions:

In a small saucepan over medium heat, combine sugar, herbs, and water until sugar is dissolved. Set aside to cool.

When the mixture has cooled, strain out herbs. Place in a pitcher with lemon juice and water; stir well to combine. Add more water or sugar, to taste, if desired. Serve over ice, garnished with fresh herbs if desired.

Jet set

Preparation time: 10 minutes

Servings: 4

Ingredients:

6 cl cucumber juice (leave the peels)

1.5 cl fresh lime juice

1.5 cl agave nectar

5 basil leaves

Directions:

Mix the basil leaves in a baking dish.

Add the other ingredients. Shake with ice.

Strain through a tea strainer with fresh ice.

Peel the cucumber. Garnish with cucumber ribbons.

Cherry lime spritz

Preparation time: 10 minutes

Servings: 4

Ingredients:

2 lime wedges

2 tbsp. freshly squeezed lime juice

2 tbsp. 100% cherry juice

2 tbsp. simple syrup (or 4 drops of liquid stevia, or to taste)

3/4 cup of your favorite sparkling water

Additional lime wedges for garnish (optional)

Directions:

Put 2 lime wedges in the bottom of the glass. Destroy the wedges with a jumbled tool.

Add lime juice, cherry juice, and sweetener of your choice and mix up more.

Pour carbonated water into the glass.

Add a few ice cubes. Garnish with additional lime wedges if desired.

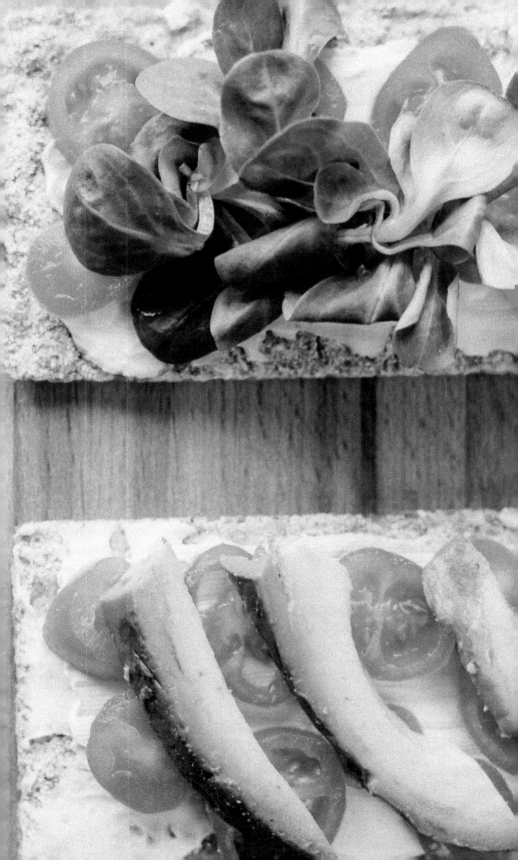

Keto Snacks for Happy Hour

No Bread Breakfast Sandwich

Preparation time: 10 minutes

Cooking Time: 15 minutes;

Servings: 2

Ingredients:

2 slices of ham

4 eggs

1 tsp tabasco sauce

3 tbsp. butter, unsalted

2 tsp grated mozzarella cheese

Seasoning:

¼ tsp salt

1/8 tsp ground black pepper

Directions:

Take a frying pan, place it over medium heat, add butter and when it melts, crack an egg in it and fry for 2 to 3 minutes until cooked to the desired level.

Transfer fried egg to a plate, fry remaining eggs in the same manner, and when done, season eggs with salt and black pepper.

Prepare the sandwich and for this, use a fried egg as a base for the sandwich, then top with a ham slice, sprinkle with a tsp of ham, and cover with another fried egg.

Place the egg into the pan, return it over low heat, and let it cook until the cheese melts.

Prepare another sandwich in the same manner and then serve.

Nutrition: 180 Calories; 15 g Fats; 10 g Protein; 1 g Net Carb; 0 g Fiber;

Scrambled Eggs with Basil and Butter

Preparation time: 5 minutes

Cooking Time: 5 minutes;

Servings: 2

Ingredients:

1 tbsp. chopped basil leaves

2 tbsp. butter, unsalted

2 tbsp. grated cheddar cheese

2 eggs

2 tbsp. whipping cream

Seasoning:

1/8 tsp salt

1/8 tsp ground black pepper

Directions:

Take a medium bowl, crack eggs in it, add salt, black pepper, cheese, and cream, and whisk until combined.

Take a medium pan, place it over low heat, add butter and when it melts, pour in the egg mixture and cook for 2 to 3 minutes until eggs have scrambled to the desired level.

When done, distribute scrambled eggs between two plates, top with basil leaves, and then serve.

Nutrition: 320 Calories; 29 g Fats; 13 g Protein; 1.5 g Net Carb; 0 g Fiber;

Bacon, and Eggs

Preparation time: 5 minutes

Cooking Time: 10 minutes;

Servings: 2

Ingredients:

2 eggs

4 slices of turkey bacon

¼ tsp salt

¼ tsp ground black pepper

Directions:

Take a skillet pan, place it over medium heat, add bacon slices in it and cook for 5 minutes until crispy.

Transfer bacon slices to a plate and set aside until required, reserving the fat in the pan.

Cook the egg in the pan one at a time, and for this, crack an egg in the pan and cook for 2 to 3 minutes or more until the egg has cooked to the desired level.

Transfer the egg to a plate and cook the other egg in the same manner.

Season eggs with salt and black pepper and then serve with cooked bacon.

Nutrition: 136 Calories; 11 g Fats; 7.5 g Protein; 1 g Net Carb; 0 g Fiber

Boiled Eggs

Preparation time: 5 minutes

Cooking Time: 10 minutes;

Servings: 2

Ingredients:

2 eggs

½ of a medium avocado

Seasoning:

¼ tsp salt

¼ tsp ground black pepper

Directions:

Place a medium pot over medium heat, fill it half full with water and bring it to boil.

Then carefully place the eggs in the boiling water and boil the eggs for 5 minutes until soft-boiled, 8 minutes for medium-boiled, and 10 minutes for hard-boiled.

When eggs have boiled, transfer them to a bowl containing chilled water and let them rest for 5 minutes.

Then crack the eggs with a spoon and peel them.

Cut each egg into slices, season with salt and black pepper, and serve with diced avocado.

Nutrition: 112 Calories; 9.5 g Fats; 5.5 g Protein; 1 g Net Carb; 0 g Fiber;

Pineapple Stew

Preparation time: 5 minutes

Cooking Time: 3 hours

Servings: 4

Ingredients:

1/2 fresh pineapple

2 cups apple juice

¼ cup of coconut sugar

Directions:

Combine all the ingredients, cook on low for 3 hours, and serve.

Nutrition: calories 282, fat 4, fiber 2, carbs 14, protein 23

Rhubarb Compote

Preparation time: 5 minutes

Cooking Time: 4 hours

Servings: 6

Ingredients:

1-pound rhubarb

1 cup of water

4 tablespoons honey

1 teaspoon vanilla extract

Directions:

Mix all the fixings, and cook on low for 4 hours, and serve.

Nutrition: calories 282, fat 4, fiber 2, carbs 14, protein 23

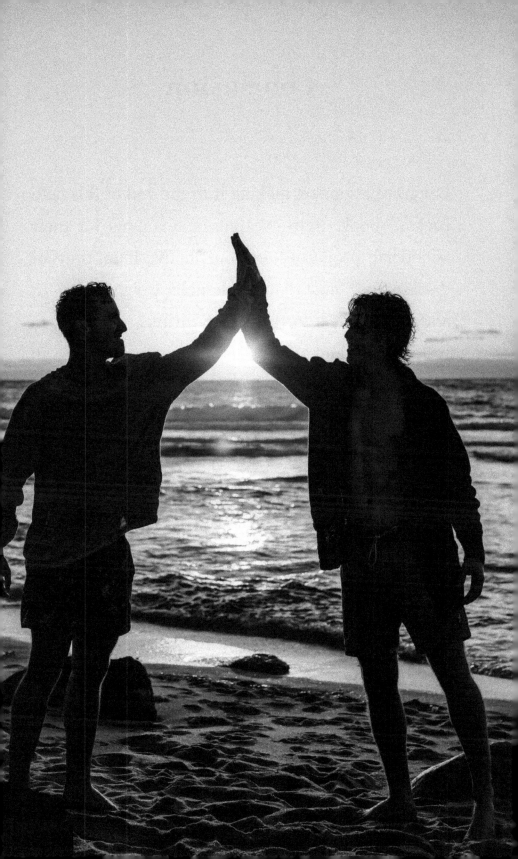

Conclusion

Congratulations on making it to the end of this keto cocktail book. Keto cocktails are famous for their beneficial properties on our body, help prevent disease and ensure considerable weight loss. In addition, thanks to these tasty drinks, our lifestyle will improve and our body will begin to eliminate all the toxins present in it. I really hope that all the cocktails we have prepared together have satisfied you and have enjoyed you.

Good luck.

Lightning Source UK Ltd.
Milton Keynes UK
UKHW022017020621
384830UK00002B/247